EARL'S SEVEN SIMPLE STEPS TO HEALING & HEALTH EXPANDED

dr.sherrillchong!!!

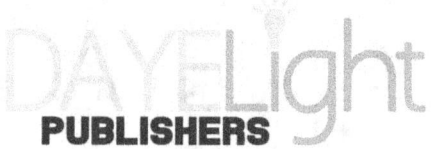

DEDICATION

To the eternal memory of a man who lived his life on earth exactly as God required… Always exhibiting and sharing the fruit of the Spirit of LOVE.

His interaction with all was:

> Joyful
> Peaceful
> Patient
> Kind
> Good
> Faithful
> Gentle and with
> Self-Control

Thank you, Father, for lending Earl to all of us, and may His legacy live on until time gives way to eternity.

Sherrill

TABLE OF CONTENTS

PROMOTED TO GLORY

Earl Constantine Chong, (Charley/Chongie) was promoted to glory on December 20, 2012.

He was pronounced dead at the Mandeville Hospital, Manchester, Jamaica; 4 hours after being taken there at 1 a.m. by his wife, Dr. Sherrill Chong, with 'shortness of breath'.

Just 16 hours before, he was doing his usual jogging on our rebounder, and showed no physical signs that this would be his last day on earth.

In this, his 72nd year, he often expressed a desire to go to be with his Father in heaven, because he had finished his course and had no desire to remain here until he became sick, and needed to be assisted by anyone.

On the night in question, he expressed the desire NOT to go to the hospital, as he would be okay. At the hospital he was put on oxygen, then nebulized, and by 3 a.m., I was given the green light by the doctors that he was now breathing normally, and I could take him home. I was very tired and nodded off to sleep while waiting, and thought it would not be wise to drive back to St. Elizabeth in that state, so requested an hour to sleep in my car before taking him home.

Life and death are in the power of the tongue, and Earl got his oft-spoken desire while I slept.

His death certificate listed pulmonary failure as a factor, and there was no 'return' of the cancer healed by God some 20 years before.

All healing comes from God. Both Earl and Sherrill experienced complete healing from cancer – Earl, larynx and prostate; and Sherrill, larynx and brain. Our lifestyle changes were not to help out God, but to honour Him in obedience to His Word to 'go thy way and sin no more'; (remember that the curse does not come without a cause); and to preserve His temple (our bodies) as best we could.

WHY THIS REPRINT?

The original book and Earl's story of healing and health has been around the world, and has positively affected the health of millions of persons. Over the past 8 years, I have received numerous requests for the booklet, and decided 6 years ago to update the materials and protocols to reflect the immense research done in the field of Kingdom Health since the book was first published. This, however, required too many changes and would not reflect the protocols that Earl actually used to reverse His negative symptoms and maintain a healthy life until his death.

I have decided instead to list some of the major changes to our protocols, the new areas of research focus, and some of the new training and empowerment programs now available.

Major Changes

Earl and I were trained some 20 years ago as *Health Ministers* at Hallelujah Acres in Shelby, North Carolina; and had adopted the *Hallelujah Diet* and lifestyle. Understandably, the training and recommendations were all using fruits, vegetables, nuts, seeds, peas, beans and grain grown in the United States of America and Northern climates. On our return to Jamaica, we started our 15-year research journey to find and develop locally-produced substitutes that were far healthier for those of us who dwell in this region. We have produced over 400 new products from locally grown produce and the number increases weekly. I list a few below.

Local Substitutes:

<u>Moringa leaves or Callaloo</u> for Barley grass – available fresh, as seedlings, powder, tea, liquids,

fertilizer, growth hormone, flocculent, animal feed, etc.,

<u>Coconut Oil for Olive Oil</u> – boiled, cold-pressed, extracted and fermented;

<u>Fresh Cane Juice</u> for Agave, Maple Syrup, Stevia, and natural cane sugar;

<u>Fresh locally-grown herbs & spices</u> for all imported herbs and spices, especially those dried, processed or extracted.

<u>Sweet Potato</u> for Irish Potato…

<u>and a plethora of local fruits, vegetables, nuts & seeds (almonds, cashew nuts, coconut, sunflower); peas & beans; and grain</u>, for all imported items in these categories.

We eliminated all locally produce items that have been genetically modified; and continue to reduce all hybrid produce and revert as much as available, to those items that are less modified. Most importantly, we have developed health and healing protocols not led by diet or nutritional changes, but by biblical principles of locating the spiritual root of all conditions which manifest in our bodies. Wherever you live across the world, try to use only locally grown food items and avoid food items imported from geographical regions far removed from your own locale; as they do not provide the optimal benefits for the healing process.

RESEARCH FOCUS

During the first three years of starting the *Earl's Juice Garden Chain,* there were dramatic testimonials of 'healings' as a result of diet changes, and my husband and I were in demand as presenters and conference speakers across the island of Jamaica and did a Caribbean Peoples tour to satisfy the interest of our people overseas. We were constantly on Radio, Television and in the newspapers… and every now and then one of our faithful customers, dropped dead; or "the cancer returned with a vengeance" and they were gone within weeks.

We returned to the drawing board, and during my doctoral studies in *Clinical Christian Counseling, I* focused on *Orthomolecular Medicine & Psychiatry.* This research focus led to additional research in what God has to say about *Neuroscience, The Enteric Nervous System, DNA*

Development, Pneumapsychosomatology, (the Spirit-Soul-Body Connection); Biblical Hermeneutics & Jewish Studies, and how we can fulfill God's original mandate to be fruitful and multiply and replenish the earth; by bringing God's Kingdom on earth as it is in heaven.

This only reinforced the following non-negotiables:

1. God created us perfect, with a self-healing body, as the dwelling place of God's Spirit. It only malfunctions when it is abused.

2. God is our healer, He sent His Word to heal us. It is only as we receive and obey His Word, that we receive healing… and it happens immediately, and permanently.

3. The removal of symptoms may occur as a result of surgery, medication, therapy, supplementation, change of diet, or a host of traditional, or non-traditional interventions. This does not in any way impact the root of diseased conditions, which are all in the spiritual realm.

This gave rise to a WAY of living that exemplifies God's intent for living in the Kingdom of God on earth as it is in heaven. This process is still evolving as daily downloads are received from God to grow in grace and the knowledge and wisdom of God to successfully live, and successfully war. Below are the main protocols that resulted from the above research.

THE 3-7-12 WAY

THE 3-7-12 WAY is a series of Kingdom Lifestyle Protocols addressing the diseases of the Spirit, Soul, and Body and providing biblical interventions that work all the time, with everyone. These Protocols identify only the root causes of all conditions, and are based on the SHEMA of God's Word.

SHMA ISRAEL, ADONAI ELOHENU ADONAI EHAD

Hear Oh Israel, The Lord Thy God is One, (and I Shall Worship Him with all my heart, my mind, my soul, my strength).

Listed on the following pages are snippets of protocols which will help those interested in walking in THE WAY that God has graciously provided for all men to experience divine health and healing.

TOXICITY ASSESSMENT

Every BODY carries a toxic load, resulting from inhalation, dermal absorption, ingestion AND injection. Unless there is regular cleansing at the cellular level, this toxic load provides an incubator for all negative health conditions. Listed below are some of the indicators of toxicity from head to toe, and while this may appear extensive, it is only a fraction of the many results of toxicity in our bodies.

Please place a tick through every condition you have ever experienced, (however mild or however long ago), then place the total number of ticks here.

_____

These results will determine the cell-cleansing program that is appropriate for restoring an optimal state of health.

Headache, numbness, pain, weakness, vomiting, nausea, confusion, vision disturbance, glaucoma, hypertension, meningitis, migraine, sinusitis, loss of balance, fainting, convulsions, loss of consciousness, itchy eyes, discharge from eyes, macular degeneration, stroke, ringing in ears, dizziness, tapeworms, discharge from ears, earache, deafness, ruptured eardrum, sudden nosebleed, mucous in nose, draining sinuses, sore mouth, dry mouth, candidiasis, cold sores, lupus, tetanus, tooth abscess, Bell's Palsy, Parkinson's disease, swelling on neck, swollen glands, German measles, goiter, lymphoma, esophageal cancer, tonsillitis, hyperthyroidism, stiffness in neck, sore throat, coughing, hoarseness, bronchitis, chicken pox, croup, hay fever, typhoid fever, influenza, pharyngitis, laryngitis, chest pain, angina aneurysm, heartburn, aortic valve disease, arteriosclerosis, coronary artery disease, hiatus hernia, pulmonary embolism, breathing difficulty, chills, asbestosis, bronchitis, lung cancer, pneumonia, wheezing, tuberculosis, anxiety, allergies, asthma, cystic fibrosis, round worms, hyperventilation, colic, whooping cough, swollen lymph nodes, breast abscess, breast cancer, mastitis, gall stones, hernia, appendicitis, liver abscess, ovarian cysts, stomach ulcer, pancreatic cancer, diarrhea, indigestion, constipation, weight loss, food poisoning, Crohn's Disease, cholera, gastritis, diverticular disease, pale fatty stools, irritable bowel syndrome, vomiting blood, stomach cancer, gastric erosion, lower back pain, kidney stones, endometriosis, sciatica, pancreatic cancer, polycystic kidney disease, osteoporosis, prolapsed spinal disc, stiffness & pain & weakness in joints, carpal tunnel syndrome, gout, bursitis, frozen shoulder, limb dislocation, osteoarthritis, spinal cord tumor, rheumatoid arthritis, tendinitis, systemic lupus, weakness in limb, leg pain & tenderness, multiple sclerosis, neuritis, leg pain & tenderness, thrombosis, varicose veins, muscular spasm, twitches, or weakness, cerebral palsy, convulsions, epilepsy, Guillain-Barre syndrome, Parkinson's, blood in feces, anal fissure, cirrhosis of the liver, hemorrhoids, rectal abscess, prolapsed or tumor, stomach ulcer, vaginal bleeding, abruptio placentae, ectopic pregnancy, fibroids, uterine or vaginal cancer, vaginal discharge, cervical cancer, gonorrhea, vaginitis, pelvic inflammatory disease, penis discharge/pain/ulceration frequent urination or with pain, syphilis, non-specific urethritis, testicular cancer, swelling or pain in testicles, skin lesions, pustules, or itching. Athlete's foot, AIDS, acne, boil, herpes, cold sores, corns & bunions, eczema, lupus, melanoma, psoriasis, ring worm, scabies, shingles, skin cancer, rosacea, yellow skin, cirrhosis of the liver, gangrene, jaundice, sickle cell anemia, pancreatic cancer, urine frequency with pain or blood, bladder stones, bladder tumor, prostate cancer or enlargement, vaginal cancer, urine retention, kidney failure, prostate gland enlargement. Dark/ strong smelling urine, cystitis, tuberculosis, behavioral changes, alcoholism, dementia, Alzheimer's, brain tumor, drug abuse, delirium, rabies, head injury, anemia, diabetes, blood poisoning, blackheads, dengue, influenza, tonsillitis, pink eye.

Note any other negative symptom/condition not mentioned above, and include in the number noted above.

DISEASE REVERSAL PROTOCOL

L isted below are the principles of Disease Reversal, which apply to any negative condition which exists in the body. All disease starts in the spirit realm, as a result of acting contrary to your best interest as revealed to you by God's Spirit to your inner man. This action creates chemical imbalances in your neurotransmitters causing them to mal-function. The following processes and the adoption of the attached CHANGE AGENTS will result in a renewed spirit, soul, and body.

STOP:

- All Flesh Foods
- All Dairy Products
- All Processed/GMO foods
- Diffuse negative emotions
- Replace stress reactions with stress responses.

CLEANSE:

- Liquid Waste
- Solid Waste
- Gaseous Waste
- Mucous Waste
- Toxic Relationships & Toxic Stress

BUILD with the 5 Elements of Life:

- Fresh Air
- Pure Water
- Direct Sunlight
- Whole Earth Foods
- PEMF's

Love, Laugh, & Live with Shalom!

CHANGE AGENTS

1. LOVE – The greatest Change Agent and the
   only motivator that engenders true change!!!

The Five Portals:

2. SOUND

3. SIGHT

4. SPEECH

5. SMELL

6. TOUCH

The Five Elements:

7. FRESH AIR

8. PURE WATER

9. SUNLIGHT

10. EARTH FOODS

11. PEMF'S (Pulsed Electro-magnetic Fields)

Earth Minerals:

12. VITAMINS

13. MINERALS

14. PROTEIN

15. CHLOROPHYLL

16. ENZYMES

Foods that Heal:

17. FRUITS

18. VEGETABLES

19. NUTS, SEEDS

20. PEAS, BEANS

21. GRAIN

Training & Empowerment

Earl Chong has always been big on training and empowerment. Wherever he saw potential, he was quick to provide the means for advancement. He was always teaching everyone to fish! In continuing this trend, I list below consultations, seminars, training programs, organizational health assessments, and soon-to-be-published writings from our current offerings.

CONSULTATIONS

Mini-Consults (30 mins)

- Weight Management

- The Ultimate Detox

- Disease Reversal

- Kingdom Family Health

- Therapeutic Farms & Gardens

- Family Financial Management

- Family Purpose, Passion & Destiny

<u>Health Audits</u> (Causes and Reversal Procedures)

6, 12 or 15 hours over 6, 12 or 15 weeks.

- Single Issue (Individual)

- Executive Health Audit Profile

- Group Health Profile

SEMINARS: Free for Churches, Schools, and Community Organizations.

- Principles of Health and Healing

- Principles of Disease Reversal

- Principles of Health Maintenance

TRAINING PROGRAMS:

Culinary Academy Classes (3 hours) also available on DVD.

Biblical Health & Healing (3 hours)

Immunology 101 (3 hours)

Immunology for Health Professionals (21 hours)

Kingdom Shift Consultants Training (21 hours)

Principles of Therapeutic Product Development (3 hours)

Workshop – Therapeutic Product Development (3-6 hrs.)

ORGANIZATIONAL HEALTH ASSESSMENTS

Assessment of the overall health of members of the group, followed by a group seminar on the Principles of Immunology, and The Seven Simple Steps to Healing & Health; suitable for companies, institutions, schools, community groups, etc.

YOU CAN... !!! Empowerment Series.

50 Publications covering the *Seven Areas of Kingdom Life!!!* The first in the series is scheduled to be in print in mid 2019; Entitled YOU CAN... Hear From God!!!

These publications will put into print the contents of approximately 200 video programs uploaded to YouTube up to 2013 plus new research since then.

Franchises will be available to operate new Earl's Juice Gardens, locally and overseas in 2020. Please indicate your interest in receiving a copy of our franchise arrangements which will be available in September 2019; by emailing us at eschong50@gmail.com indicating your parish/country of preference.

Below is the reprint of the original "EARLS SEVEN SIMPLE STEPS TO HEALING & HEALTH" which was written by Earl Chong and David Campbell. and published by Earl's Juice Garden Limited.

EARL'S SEVEN SIMPLE STEPS

TO

HEALING & HEALTH

Following is the reprint of this booklet in its original form.

INTRODUCTION

Before I learned so much about health I went through a crisis in my life. I had cancer and was told I was going to die. This is my story:

In 1992 I was diagnosed with cancer of the larynx. I spent over $3M (JA) on the best treatment available in Florida, and within a few months I learned that the cancer was still spreading.

I returned to Jamaica, convinced by the expert's verdict that I was really only going home to die. That same day in prayer I felt God's reassurance that my time had not yet come; but as time went by my condition grew worse. Within four months I was unable to speak.

At 4 a.m., six months after my treatment, I awoke with the sense that the Holy Spirit was telling me to worship God. As I did, I was led to Exodus

23:25: "And you shall serve the Lord your God, and he shall bless your bread and water. And I will take sickness away from the midst of you." At that moment, on my knees in prayer, my voice returned. The following year (1994) I was given the book "Why Christians Get Sick" by Rev. Dr. George Malkmus, who himself had recovered from cancer through nutrition and lifestyle changes. I read the book in one night, and began to make a few adjustments. However, it was not until one last trip to the doctor that I finally made a complete change. It was 1995, when I received the diagnosis that I now had prostate cancer. I simply decided "no more doctor", and walked away from the conventional medical treatment, making a full commitment to a more natural path.

My first step was to go on a 40-day juice fast, only drinking fresh vegetable and fruit juices and a minimal quantity of raw food. Since then I have maintained an 85% raw diet (only 15% cooked food in my daily intake). I chose natural, unrefined, plant based food (no meat or animal products) and regularly consume "Barleymax" (an all natural supplement), as well as vegetable juices and pure water.

To this day my cancer has not returned and I enjoy better health than ever before. My wife Sherrill and I started a health food shop; Earl's Juice Garden (now Earl's Garden), to encourage more people towards making the right choices for their own health.

Having been diagnosed with cancer twice in my life and recovered to **better health than ever before**, I feel it is my duty to share the simple steps that led to my healing with anyone who is willing to hear them. That is the reason I have written this booklet; to define the most important things we should all understand about our health, and share how to apply this knowledge in daily life.

My Philosophy

Health is a popular topic at the moment, with endless new programmes, diet supplements, articles in the newspaper (etc. etc.) and all of them claiming to have "the new-found secret". The problem with all this hype is that it leaves people confused about what to believe and what not to believe. There seems to be a different "expert" to prove every different theory we hear, so how do we know which one to trust?

In my own search for understanding I have read books by people with a very wide range of ideas, the more I have read the more I have become convinced that health is **very simple**. Some of the advice I have read makes health so complicated that I simply do not accept it. So to help you understand my philosophy of health I have summed it up in four points:

1. I believe that God is trustworthy. Therefore a natural diet and lifestyle will automatically lead to good health. I trust what grows from the **garden** which is why I believe people can trust the natural products sold in Earl's Garden.

2. I believe that health is a **choice**, not just a chance. Because of this, one of the most important things is an accurate understanding of the body and how it works. When people have a better understanding, they can make better choices and experience better health.

3. I believe that the basis of health is the **cells**. **Every cell** in the human body is replaced over time, and the nutrition we give the cells for replenishment is what determines our health. The **only** materials for building cells come to the body from the *air we breathe, the liquid we drink and the food we eat.* If these are "good" materials we will have healthy cells, otherwise we will not. Fresh

nutrients are carried to the cells by the lymphatic system, which [unlike blood circulation] has no pump; it relies on physical movement to do its job. The lymph also removes toxins. So an active life and a healthy diet are **utterly essential** for good health.

4. I believe that health is a **complete** condition. I do not believe in treating isolated complaints, as these are usually only symptoms of a greater problem. Sickness really has **only 3 causes**: deficiency (not having enough of a vital nutrient in the body) toxins (having too much of a harmful substance in the body) and stress (facing or attempting challenges that you don't have the resources for). If we eliminate these three causes we can **never be sick**. That is why I recommend a change in the entire lifestyle, rather than following an unnatural lifestyle and just adding a few healthy "supports".

Benefits

Some people seem to believe that their diet and lifestyle does not affect their health but also their whole experience of life. I have seen nutrition literally save lives, including my own, but I want to clarify here what the realistic benefits are that can be gained through my seven simple steps.

Immediate Benefits:

Firstly, you just feel better.

We all know how irritable, withdrawn and groggy we feel when we have a cold. When your body is healthy it is exactly the opposite. Stress will be reduced, and you will feel more alive and alert. Many studies show a correlation between prolonged depression and poor nutrition. Obviously, emotional trauma will affect whatever you eat, but taking steps to look after your health will improve your mood. By *the way, if you make a radical change in your diet the first thing you may experience is feeling a lot worse! Usually this will be manifested in headaches, strange muscle aches and drowsiness that lasts for 3 to 5 days. That is simply caused by your body detoxifying and cleansing itself. After this you will feel fairly normal, and may not feel much better for 2 weeks. However, in just 3 weeks you will be feeling MUCH better, and within 6 weeks you will feel so much better you will probably never want to return to your old lifestyle. It is important that you know this so that you don't give up on the second day.)*

You get sick less frequently.

Good nutrition boosts the immune system, and un-nutritious food burdens it. As a result, you will be able to avoid sicknesses that others would not avoid, and if ever you do become ill you will recover much more quickly.

You have more energy and look better.

Your energy level will be higher. It becomes easier to stay motivated and to achieve a healthy weight.

You think better.
This will include better concentration, a better memory, better spatial awareness and even better sleep.

Long Term Benefits:

You age slower.

With a healthy lifestyle, you are guaranteed to stay active and mentally alert far longer. I don't think I can make this point strong enough. *You* can be very healthy into old age; if you do something about it *now*.

You are much less likely to have heart failure or cancer.

Seeing that these two conditions account for approximately 60% of the deaths in the western world, it is worth knowing how they can be avoided. The evidence is overwhelming that heart failure and cancer are predominantly caused by **how we live.** Yes, some people have a hereditary makeup that means they are more likely to get some form of cancer; but that chance can be

radically reduced through proper nutrition and a healthy life. Once again, it was nutrition and adopting a healthy lifestyle that saved my own life from cancer.

You are much less likely to get most serious illnesses.

It is a sweeping statement I know, but there is documented evidence that nutrition can be used to help prevent and also treat all of the following: Diabetes, osteoporosis, sciatica, Alzheimer's, anaemia, gall stones, cataracts, asthma, allergies, irregular heartbeats, multiple sclerosis, Parkinsons, infertility, gout, arthritis, fibromyalgia…and the list goes on. There are endless testimonies of people with all sorts of prolonged illnesses, who experienced a dramatic recovery after changing their diets.

With all these benefits within your reach, I encourage you to take these seven steps very seriously and **make a change** in the way you live. The steps are very simple so I will now explain them:

My Seven Simple Steps to Healing and Health

Meditation

I have deliberately put this first because man should seek first the Kingdom of God and all things shall be added to him (Matt 6:33). What I mean by meditation is two things; worship and prayer. Man is created to worship God; therefore the most important function of man is to worship. If he does not worship God he will worship something else. Because God's heart is to give man the very best, whenever we worship anything other than God we are sacrificing the best thing for our lives, and as a consequence; our health. God is source and man is resource, and prayer is showing your dependence on a greater source than yourself for your life. Without it we shall never have the resources for true inner peace and fulfillment and therefore outer health. I recommend that everyone starts the day with 30 minutes to an hour of meditation.

Fresh Air

Fresh air is a *fundamental* building block for healthy cells. Every single function of the cells requires oxygen, and sickness cannot live in a properly oxygenated body.

However, the air we need is fresh air, something that is becoming harder and harder to come by. Once again plants hold the key as they produce fresh oxygen. Try to spend some time in an area with dense vegetation on a regular basis, try and get your exercise in that sort of environment. I would recommend that everyone take time 2 or 3 times a day, to breathe deeply for at least one minute in a clean environment.

Pure Water

The human body is over 70% water, and the brain is over 80% water. We need pure water for every single bodily function, yet most "drinking" water is so chlorinated and otherwise contaminated it is a serious health risk (by which I mean *very* serious).

The best options (if possible) is to have a high quality filter fitted to your main supply or buy pure drinking water (we sell both filters and pure water at Earl's Garden). We also need to drink a lot more water than most people are accustomed to. The most widely accepted recommendation for drinking water is 6 to 8 glasses per day (a glass being 8oz). This can equally be consumed as fresh or undiluted fruit or vegetable juice, which has the benefits of providing us with essential nutrients.

Tea and coffee both cause dehydration so they would not count in the same way. By simply drinking two glasses on waking, and then 30 minutes before every meal it is easy to get into this habit. It is best to drink during the day rather than at night so that you don't have to take endless trips to the bathroom when you could be sleeping.

It is also better not to drink while you eat because this only dilutes the digestive juices in your stomach.

Nutrition

Our food should satisfy our body's needs rather than our greedy appetites. In fact as soon as you start to eat the kinds of foods your body requires the hunger pangs for other foods will disappear. This is because you have finally given your body exactly what it was designed to receive from food. The five most important ingredients for health are vitamins, minerals, enzyme, protein and chlorophyll. We all know about the necessity of vitamins, minerals and protein, but enzymes and chlorophyll are often forgotten. Every single chemical reaction in the body needs enzymes as a catalyst. However, the body only has a limited supply and unless we eat food rich in live enzymes, health will be compromised. Enzymes are only found on living food such as raw fruit and raw vegetables. Cooking destroys them.

Chlorophyll gets rid of dead cells in the body, as well as being a natural energy source. Chlorophyll is a product of plant photosynthesis. It has a molecular structure that is almost identical to haemoglobin in human blood so consuming foods high in chlorophyll will improve the health of the blood, the process of replenishing cells and therefore total well-being.

These are the most important things to do in order to achieve a healthy nutritional intake.

Eat more vegetables than any other food. All vegetables are excellent for health, and green vegetables are especially good. Vegetable juices are an excellent way of adding more essential nutrients to your diet (especially carrot juice) Buying a juicer is one of the healthiest investments you can make.

Eat plenty of fruit. Fruits are a rich supply of vitamins, antioxidants and fibre, and should also be eaten daily. Excessive fruit can be harmful because of the sugar content, so aim for fruit to make up about 15% of your daily intake. Fruit juices are also rich in vitamins, but they need to be fresh, *not* the preserved, sweetened juices as sold in most shops. Get plenty of fibre. Fibre is found in almost all vegetables, brown rice, whole grains, potato (especially with the skin on) and fruit like apple and peaches (also with the skin). Fibre helps move food through the intestines, and is essential for healthy digestion. Low fibre intake and cancer have strong links, as well as links to prolonged depression.

Eat mostly raw food. Most vegetables can be eaten raw, as can nuts, seeds, fruit, dried fruit etc. Even some carbohydrates may be eaten raw. Raw food has a host of benefits, mainly due to the fact that all the nutrients and enzymes are taken into the body rather than lost or killed in the cooking process. Boiling vegetables for 10 minutes means the water (that we throw away) contains more nutrients than the vegetables we eat.

Sunshine

Sunshine is a tremendous gift from God that is not only pleasant but gives us numerous health benefits. Sunlight on the skin is the only way the body can resource the production of vitamin D, which is essential for making use of calcium. Studies also show that proper (not excessive) exposure to the sun lowers blood pressure, reduces the heart resting rate, balances the production of hormones, strengthens the immune system, lowers blood sugar levels, increases cardiac output and increases stress tolerance levels. Because of the dangers of excessive exposure to the sun and the depleted ozone layer it is best to spend time in the sun during the cooler parts of the day.

Exercise

There are so many reasons our bodies need to be active, there are endless books that deal with nothing else. No matter what people eat, regular exercise cannot be neglected if people want to be healthy. It strengthens the heart, helps the lungs function, enables the lymph to circulate, detoxifies the body (there are numerous contaminants that cannot be excreted by other means than sweat) improves circulation and enhances a positive outlook on life. Without exercise we lose all these benefits, which makes us far more susceptible to disease and ill health. Try to build some form of exercise in to your daily routine (the more vigorous the better!)

Rest

We live in an accelerated world, and it is killing us. We must re-learn the importance of rest and take time to relax daily. Eating should be a relaxing experience and not on the run between more hurried tasks. Eating on the run has two serious problems; 1) We don't chew our food well enough (nutritionists estimate that at least 80% of people do not chew their food sufficiently) which gives the digestive system more work.

The body stays in what is known as the "fight or flight" mode. The central nervous system is all hyped up and ready for action, which puts the digestive system on hold to preserve energy for whatever the action may be. Eating in this state will make digestion ineffective, wasting whatever nutrients your body could have used.

Also a good night's sleep is essential for the body and the mind to function well. It is not possible to get the benefits of good sleep by sleeping for a short time and then "catching up" by napping in the day. Healthy habits will give you better sleep, but you can't sleep well if you don't go to bed! Over sleeping can be just as damaging, so the healthiest habit is getting 7 or 8 hours of regular, quality sleep every night.

Things To Avoid

As I have mentioned, there is so much nutrient- deficient, processed and really quite dangerous "food" in our common diets that we need to avoid some common "foods" if we want to stay healthy.

White Flour

White flour contains almost nothing of nutritional value whatsoever. It also sticks to the walls of the intestines; disrupting digestion. It really is NOT good food and should be avoided altogether. Whole wheat flour can be used instead in almost all recipes, but beware of "whole wheat" bread and other products because most of them are simply white flour with some bran added.

Refined Sugar

Refined sugar (white sugar) is a simple carbohydrate, so it is absorbed straight into the bloodstream, requiring minimal digestion. It causes a sudden increase in blood sugar level, so the body then reacts by releasing insulin, which reduces the blood sugar level so effectively that within 30 minutes you have less energy than before. Refined sugar is linked to many behavioural problems (especially in children) and is the biggest cause of lack of energy. It also represses the immune system, making people more prone to sickness. Soft drinks, cakes, sweets, chocolate and ice cream which are rich in refined sugar, should be eliminated from the diet.

Salt, Additives and Preservatives

Sodium is a necessary part of our diet, but table salt is an inorganic form of sodium chloride that the body cannot break down or absorb. The sodium is never separated from the chloride in order to become a useable nutrient. Salt enhances the flavor of foods which is why it is so common, but it should be used in small quantities (sea salt is less harmful because it is in an organic form). Salt is used in most packaged foods, in large quantities. Too much table salt contributes to congestive heart failure, fluid retention and high blood pressure among other health problems. Other preservatives contribute to the same conditions, while additives (E numbers etc.) are utterly inorganic substances that the body cannot benefit from, and struggles to dispose of.

Caffeine

Caffeine is a powerful stimulant, forcing the body into "fight or flight" mode. This slows digestion and prevents essential nutrients from being absorbed. It also has a direct impact on the immune system, causing it to be less effective.

Fat

Fat is an essential part of a healthy diet, but once again these need to be *naturally occurring* fats, and they need to be consumed sparingly. Excessive fat in the diet is the *main* cause of high cholesterol (*not* cholesterol in the diet) and therefore heart disease. Hydrogenated fats (man-made like margarine) are so hard for the body to pass through the body that some nutritionists label them as "the most dangerous foodstuff in the modern market". You can get more than adequate supply of essential fats from raw seeds (sunflower seeds, flax seeds & sesame seeds especially), nuts and avocado.

Animal Products

Excessive animal protein is *directly linked* to the probability of developing several cancers. Also, many of the modern production methods of meat cause nutritionists to doubt its safety. Even fish are caught from such highly polluted waters that there is a concern about health risks. Meat definitely is **not** a necessary part of a healthy diet if you know what else to eat. Legumes (beans), green vegetables and nuts are rich in protein, and essential fatty acids are found in seeds. I would recommend a diet that is completely free from animal products, but for those who cannot accept this, it is definitely worthwhile keeping meat consumption to a minimum and eating far more vegetables and unrefined plant – based food.

It is proven that people who make a **more drastic change** to these habits are those who will be **more likely** to keep up with the change. This is mainly because they see such radical results that they do not want to return to life as before. The ideal diet is 85% raw, with vegetables as the highest percentage (35 – 45%), followed by fruit (up to 15%), and the remaining can be raw seeds, nuts, cooked vegetables, cooked grains and oils (not hydrogenated, man – made oils).

A DAY IN THE LIFE

These are some general guidelines for those who want to start a healthy lifestyle.

For each time of day, pick one or two of the items from the list. Those with serious illnesses will need to be more extreme and follow a healing diet (as described on page 49).

ON WAKING:

- 2 glasses of pure water/ coconut water / ginger tea

BREAKFAST:

- Barleymax: 1 teaspoon dry under tongue or in pure water/ a fruit shake / vegetable juice

MID MORNING SNACK:

- Vegetable juice/fresh fruit

LUNCH: (preferably all uncooked)

- Barleymax 20 – 30 minutes before huge salad / raw vegetables / fruit/ soup/rye or whole wheatbread

EARLY AFTERNOON SNACK:

- Piece of fruit/dried fruits/nuts or seeds

MID AFTERNOON:

- Exercise (this is the ideal time for exercise)
- Barleymax then shower

LATE AFTERNOON:

- Juice (Carrot/apple/green)

SUPPER:

- Large salad / blended salad (like cold soup) /raw vegetable starter then main meal (carbohydrate, protein and vegetables)

It is much better to eat your main meal at least 3 – 4 hours before you go to bed, and then have a *small* snack if you are hungry later on. (Eating a banana late at night can help you sleep.) Remember to drink eight glasses of water each day.

Healing Diet:

This diet is only for times of recovery and recuperation from serious illnesses, or as a short-term period of cleansing, not for everyday life.

2 glasses of pure water / Coconut water

Through the day:

1 glass fruit juice
4 glasses Barleymax
7 glasses of vegetable juice (find out best juice for your condition from any branch of Earl's Garden).
- Carrot
- Carrot / Apple
- Carrot / Cucumber / Beet
- Carrot / String Beans / Celery
- Carrot / Beet / Callaloo
- Potato / Pumpkin / Tomato

1 or 2 vegetable salads or blended salads (like a cold soup)

In order to get the full benefits of this diet the following are recommended:

- Clear the bowels
- Get daily exposure to sunshine
- Clear the lymphatic channels (through a lymph draining massage, rebounding or a chi machine).
- Try to deal positively with negative emotions.

CONCLUSION

I hope you have found this booklet helpful and interesting. My prayer is that it would have inspired you to **make a change** in your life and **choose health.**

Though these steps are simple, you may need guidance and motivation to follow them. At Earl's Garden, we offer courses on healthy living, and will help people get started. Because these steps saved my life and keep me in wonderful health – I would recommend them to anyone. Your health is well worth the effort.

Visit Earl's Garden For:

- ✓ Natural Juices
- ✓ Health food restaurant
- ✓ Delivery Service
- ✓ Fruit and Vegetables
- ✓ Healthy baked snacks
- ✓ Health products
- ✓ Books and Videos
- ✓ Pure water
- ✓ Groceries
- ✓ Health Consultation
- ✓ & much more

ABOUT THE AUTHOR

Dr. Sherrill Elisabeth Chong is co-founder of Earl's Juice Gardens Health Stores, along with her late husband Earl Constantine Chong.

From childhood, Sherrill has been passionate about experiencing and expressing all that God created her to BE. The ultimate perpetual student, she has pursued post graduate studies in Clinical Christian Counseling Psychology, Biblical Hermeneutics & Jewish Studies, Neuroscience and the Bible, and Pneumapsychosomatology; for the purpose of empowering others to successfully live in God's Kingdom on earth, as it is in heaven.

Join me in making your life, family and environment, like heaven on earth.

Call: (876) 819-3377
Email: dr.sherrill@yahoo.com
Web: www.celebratelife.me
View SCTV at Reggaetoreggae.com
Available on Amazon.com